Natural Skin Secrets

80+ Homemade Beauty Treatments
and Skin Care Recipes

Angela Boket

Disclaimer

The recipes in this book are for informational use only. Nothing in this hook is a substitute for medical advice. If you have a skin condition or health problem, consult your personal health care provider.

Avoid using any of these products if you are allergic to it.

Table of Contents

Introduction

While the woman is young she usually pays no attention to such trifles as a small wrinkle on her forehead or near her mouth. She will just make up her lips and eyelashes, run the powder brush along her nose and cheeks, and feel attractive or even irresistible.

However, as soon as the lady turns 30, her life becomes impossible: she runs around beauty parlors, consults cosmetologists, and taking care of her skin takes so long that you have to wonder when she finds the time for anything else.

Each of us would love to preserve our beauty until an old age, and we become very upset looking into the mirror and seeing new wrinkles on our face.

Small creases and bags under the eyes, an unexpected jowl and other cosmetic facial defects make women bite their lips and spend fortunes on creams, lotions, facial masks – which often only make things worse.

So what can you do? First of all, not give in to panic. The first wrinkles do not at all mean that the woman has to accept the inevitable. Your inner charm never ages, and as for your appearance, you can "touch it up" or even get it back with specially selected creams, facial masks, lotions and other makeup preparations or skincare conditioners. In this book we will speak about facial masks.

What You Must Know

Skin is human or animal outer covering. It is a complex formation performing a wide variety of functions. An adult person's skin area covers from $1^1/_2$ to 2 m². 1 cm² contains about 6 million cells. Skin has different thickness and structure in different parts of the body.

Skin is composed of three main layers. The outermost – epidermis, or cuticle, consists of squamous cells which die off and peel off all the time. Skin cells are fully replaced within 26 to 28 days. The thickness of the epidermis depends on the executive function. On the hands and feet it is coarser. It communicates our body with the environment and consists of five layers: a base, styloid, granular, shining, and horny. Epidermis is covered by a surface membrane which is formed by mixing of sebum and perspiration. The next layer is dermis, or skin, which is actually formed by connective tissue.

The dermis is composed of two layers: the superficial (papillary) and deeper (reticular). And the deepest layer of skin which is called hypodermis, which consists of connective tissue fibers and fat tissue that protects organs beneath it from mechanical damage and temperature extremes.

Skin also contains two types of glands: sudoriferous and sebaceous. Sudoriferous glands are located along the whole surface of the body but they are mostly concentrated in joint flexions. A large variety of sebaceous glands are located in the centre of the face, on the back, in the upper part of the bust, but not on the palms and the soles of the feet.

Skin has several protective functions: it prevents negative influence of the environment on the human body, takes part in metabolism, plays the key role in touch, discharge processes and heat regulation.

Skin is one of the main indicators of health. There are several factors improving its condition: a balanced diet, daily care, normal gastrointestinal tract performance, sufficient sleep, self-composure, physical exercise.

Facial skin can be roughly divided into three types, each with their own peculiarities. The main types are normal, dry and oily. Besides, there is combination, aging and sensitive skin types. Let us speak about each of them in more detail.

Normal skin type is probably the least common. It is smooth, quite elastic, with even texture and almost imperceptible pores. This mat skin is moist enough but, given wrong care, may become dry or, which is more common, oily.

Dry skin type looks very attractive at a young age, it has mat texture with unnoticeable pores and appears to be smooth and tender but with age and given wrong care, it starts to wrinkle. This skin type requires moistening and nutrition.

Oily skin type has an orange peel texture: rough, with large pores and comedones (black heads). Often oily skin has a sickly gray shade.

Combination skin type is the most common one. It is oily in the centre of the face, the T-zone (the forehead, nose and chin) while the sides are either dry or normal. Its care becomes more challenging than for one of the main types: the oily zones require oily skin type care while the dry ones need their own corresponding care.

Each person acquires aging skin type with age. It is quite easy to describe: the skin becomes covered in wrinkles, it is not moist enough (aging skin is usually dry), the texture is mat, with pigment spots.

Sensitive skin is subject to various irritations. Both oily and dry skin can be sensitive. Affected by warmth, cold or wind it becomes red and inflamed. Often it peels off, especially if the makeup preparations are selected wrongly.

It is quite easy to do a home-test for your skin type. A cosmetologist will, obviously, do it more successfully but there is a series of tests fit to do at home.

"FIVE SPOTS" – CLASSIC TEST

You will need some cigarette tissue (but even a paper tissue will do). Before doing this test you should clean your face with water and soap and then wait for one or two hours so that the natural texture of the skin could recover. Put the tissue on your face and press it lightly. If the skin is oily, you will see 5 oily spots: in the forehead, nose, chin and cheek zones. Normal and combination skin types leave 3 spots, in the centre of the tissue: the forehead, nose and chin zones. Dry skin does not leave any oily spots at all, just like normal skin disposed to dryness.

SENSITIVE SKIN TEST

Sensitive skin can also be determined by a test.

The procedure is quite simple. Clean your face, sharpen your pencil and make a light line on your face. If the red trace does not disappear for several minutes, your skin is sensitive.

ROTARY-COMPRESSIVE TEST

This test will allow you to determine how elastic your skin is. Put your thumb to your cheek, press lightly and make a rotary movement. If you feel resistance to the movement and pressure, your skin is elastic. If the fan-shaped movements make wrinkles appear and disappear at once, the elasticity is not strong enough, and you should pay more attention to the skin nutrition. If light pressure immediately causes numerous wrinkles, you have the aging skin type.

Ingredients for the masks and their properties

CAMMOMILE can be used both fresh and dried; added to the bath and steam bath, used for compresses and infusions.

HONEY softens and smoothes the skin.

EGGS. The yokes nourish the skin, the whites tighten and lighten it.

PORRIDGE cleans and softens the skin. It is a perfect base for scrubs and nutritious masks.

SALT adds vitality, removes the extra liquid and saturates the skin with minerals. A salt bath prepares the skin for other treatments.

TURMERIC is a fine base for masks and scrubs. Has a healing effect.

SUGAR can be added to body scrubs to polish and soften the skin.

CUCUMBERS have moistening, cooling and slightly astringent effects.

OIL. Sunflower oil is used for massage and nutritious masks.

GRAPES moisturize and soften the skin.

PEACHES smooth and soften the skin.

COWBERRIES & BILBERRIES narrow pores.

STRAWBERRIES moisturize the skin.

BLACKCURRENTS narrow pores.

RASPBERRIES moisturize the skin.

APRICOTS have a soothing effect.

AUBERGINES AND EGGPLANTS moisturize inflamed skin.

BANANS moisturize, smooth and soften the skin.

LEMONS narrow pores (juice of other fruit is always added to lemon juice because the latter is particularly strong).

CUCUMBERS smooth and lighten the skin, narrow pores.

CARROT AND APPLE mask moisturizes and smoothes the skin.

TOMATO mask is recommended for oily skin of an earthy color.

GREEN PEAS smooth and freshen the skin to add it a mat shade.

Cosmetic face masks

Before applying any facial mask you should keep several rules in mind:

1) Remove all the make-up, clean your face deeply and apply the mask only afterwards.
2) Prepare the mask directly before its use.
3) Apply the mask avoiding the eye area. You may cover your eyelids with cotton pads damped in strong tea or chamomile infusion.
4) Never leave the mask longer than necessary; otherwise it will do more damage than good.
5) Before applying the mask you should lie down and relax your facial muscles as much as possible.
6) You can apply the mask with a brush or a cotton pad. The movements should go from the chin to the temples, from the upper lip to the lobe of the ear, from the wings of nose and centre of the forehead to the temples.

Oily Skin Type Masks

Oily skin type masks should be scrubbing and tightening. Oily skin type needs deep cleaning more often than aging or dry ones. Women often think that oily skin does not require nutrition or moisturizing, but it is a wrong assumption. This skin type does not receive enough nutrients, therefore nutritious facial masks are necessary for this skin type as well.

The ingredients for oily skin type masks are different from other facial mask types. Oily skin is characterized by larger pores and sebaceous glands inflammation. Therefore the masks should contain tightening and disinfecting components.

Egg White Whitening Mask

Ingredients:
1 egg white
10 g of kaolin (white clay)
1/2 teaspoon of alum
1/2 teaspoon of starch

Instructions:
1. Mix all these ingredients.
2. Apply on the face for 30 minutes, rinse with warm water.

Lemon mask

Ingredients:
1 lemon
100 g of vodka

Instructions:
1. Lemon crush, leave for 6-10 days in vodka and strain.
2. Dampen a cloth, put on your face.
3. Do not rinse.

Purifying mustard Mask

Ingredients:
1 teaspoon of dry mustard
2 teaspoons of vegetable oil

Instructions:
1. Mix all products.
2. Apply on face for 5 minutes and if you will feel a burning sensation, rinse with cool water before the specified time.
3. Then rub into skin cream containing menthol.

Mask from wheat and honey

Ingredients:
2 tablespoons of wheat flour
1 tablespoon of apple cider vinegar
1 teaspoon of honey
1 teaspoon of lemon juice

Instructions:
1. Mix all products.
2. Apply on the face on half an hour.
3. Rinse with cool water.

Egg white mask

Ingredients:
1 egg white
1 tablespoon of corn or oat flour

Instructions:
1. Shake up the egg white. Mix it with corn or oat flour.
2. Apply on the face.
3. Once dry, shake by dry swab.

Mask from yeast and sour cream

Ingredients:
20 g of yeast

Sour cream or milk

Instructions:
1. Mix the yeast with sour cream or milk before formation of porridge.
2. Apply on the face for 20 minutes.
This mask dries and softens skin

The mask from fresh yeast and hydrogen peroxide

Ingredients:
20 g of yeast
A few drops of lemon juice
3% hydrogen peroxide

Instructions:
1. Mix the yeast with a few drops of lemon juice and a small amount of 3% hydrogen peroxide.
2. Whisk all ingredients to the foam.
3. Apply on the face for 5-20 minutes.

The mask from honey and flour with egg white

Ingredients:
1 egg white
1 teaspoon of honey and flour

Instructions:
1. Beat the egg white, add honey and mix.
2. Add the flour to obtain a mass in the form of a thick porridge.
3. Apply on the face for 20 minutes.

Mask from the egg white and lemon

Ingredients:
1 egg white
1 teaspoon of lemon juice

Instructions:

1. Beat the protein to the thick foam.
2. Add the lemon juice.
3. Apply on the face for 20 minutes.

The skin after this mask will get a matte finish.

Mask from cottage cheese, sour cream and egg white

Ingredients:
100 g of cottage cheese
1 tablespoon of sour cream
1 egg white

Instructions:
1. Mix cottage cheese with sour cream and beaten egg white to form a thick porridge.
2. Apply on the face for 15-20 minutes.
This mask is very useful for the skin inflamed after suntan.

Cocoa Mask

Ingredients:
1/2 tablespoon of milk
1/3 cup of cocoa powder
1/4 cup of honey
4 tablespoon of oatmeal

Instructions:
1. Mix all the ingredients in a bowl.
2. Apply to face and don't forget to avoid eye area.
3. Gently massage in a circular motion.
4. Leave it for 15 – 20 minutes, rinse with warm water.
This mask is grate for moisturizing and cleansing your oily skin.

Yogurt Mask

Ingredients:
1 tablespoon of brewer's yeast
Plain yogurt

Instructions:
1. Mix all the ingredients to make a thin mixture.
2. Apply it thoroughly into all the oily areas on your face and leave for 15 – 20 minutes.
3. Rinse with warm water and apply cream.

Mask for Acne Skin

Ingredients:
1 chopped, ripe tomato
1 teaspoon of lemon juice
1 tablespoon of instant oatmeal or rolled oats.

Instructions:
1. Puree all the ingredients in a blender. If mixture seems too runny add more oats.
2. Apply on the face for 10 – 15 minutes.
3. Rinse with warm water.

Oatmeal mask

Ingredients:
1/2 boiled apple
1 teaspoon of honey
2 teaspoons of ground oatmeal

Instructions:
1. Mix all ingredients until you get an uniform mixture
2. Apply on the face for 10 minutes and wash carefully afterward.

The oatmeal is good for pimples, it also absorb the excess oil on the skin. The acids in the apple remove the dead skin cells and clean the pores. The honey works as an antibacterial ointment that destroys bacterium that can cause infections.

Tomato mask

Ingredients:

1 medium tomato
½ of a lemon
½ spoon of fresh lemon juice

Instructions:
1. Mash one medium tomato.
2. Add scraped peel from half of a lemon and a half of spoon of fresh lemon juice.
3. Apply on the face, except near the eyes.
4. Leave for 10 minutes and then rinse with lukewarm water.

This mask tightens the pores.

Walnut mask

Ingredients:
2 spoons of ground walnut
1/2 mashed cucumber
2 spoons of yogurt
1 spoon of squashed yeast

Instructions:
1. Mix it all up.
2. Apply on clean face for 20 minutes.
3. Rinse with lukewarm water.

Strawberry Lemon Mask

Ingredients:
1 teaspoon of lemon juice
2 egg whites
2 teaspoons of honey
1 cup of strawberries

Instructions:
1. Blend all the above ingredients .
2. Apply to face, leave on for 10 minutes.
3. Wash face with lukewarm water.
4. Pat your face dry with a soft towel.

Strawberry Butter Mask

Ingredients:

1 tablespoon of unsalted butter, softened
1 large strawberry, mashed

Instructions:

1. Beat both the above ingredients together.
2. Apply to face, leave on for 10 minutes.
3. Wash face with lukewarm water.
4. Pat your face dry with a soft towel.

Lemon Butter Mask

Ingredients:

1 tablespoon of unsalted butter, softened
1 teaspoon of lemon juice

Instructions:

1. Beat both the above ingredients together.
2. Apply to face for 10 minutes.
3. Wash face with lukewarm water.
3. Pat your face dry with a soft towel.

Egg White Mask

Ingredients:

1 egg white
6 drops witch hazel
6 drops lemon juice

Instructions:

1. Whisk in a bowl the egg white until stiff peaks form, add the rest of ingredients listed above.

2. Apply to the face and avoid your eyes. Leave on for 10 minutes, or let dry, and rinse off with lukewarm water.

3. Pat your face dry with a soft towel.

Carrot Mask

Ingredients:

2 to 3 large carrots

2 tablespoons of honey
1 tablespoon of olive oil
2 tablespoons of water (or as needed)

Instructions:
1. Peal the skin off the carrots. Boil the carrots until soft and tender and then mash until creamy.

2. Add the honey and olive oil to the carrots and mix until all ingredients are completely blended.

3. If the mixture appears too thick, such as a cookie dough, add the water as needed until it is a smooth, creamy consistency like pancake batter.

4. Cleanse and rinse your face with warm water before applying the mask to open your pores.

5. Apply the mask to your face and allow it to set for 20 minutes or until it begins to harden.

6. Rinse your face gently with warm water and dry.

7. Reapply the mask at least once a week to make sure your skin maintains a beautiful, healthy glow.

Banana and Honey Face Mask

Ingredients:
1 banana (ripe bananas work best)
1 tablespoon of honey

Instructions:
1. Use a fork to mash the banana. Add the honey and stir until smooth.

2. Apply to face with fingertips in a circular motion. Let it sit on your face for 15 minutes.

3. Rinse thoroughly.

Clay Mask

Ingredients:
1 tablespoon green clay
Water

Instructions:
1. Mix green clay with enough water to make a yogurt-like paste.
2. Use your fingers to spread the mask on your face.
3. Let it sit for 15 minutes before rinsing.

Green clay draws impurities from the skin and absorbs extra oil.

Gram flour face mask

Ingredients:
2 tablespoons of gram flour
A pinch of turmeric
1 tablespoon of sandalwood powder
2 tablespoons of fresh milk

Instructions:
1. Mix all the ingredients to make a smooth and fine paste
2. Wash the face with luke warm water before applying it
3. Pat it dry
4. Now apply the face pack using a soft brush
5. Wait and relax for 10-15 minutes
6. Once the face pack gets dried up, moisten the face with little amount of water and then remove it using wet cotton or sponge
7. Wipe the face with a soft towel and apply a moisturizer.

Lemon Tomato Mask

Ingredients:
1 over-ripe tomato; inside scooped and mashed
1 teaspoon of lemon juice
1 teaspoon of instant oatmeal
Instructions:
1. Puree all ingredients in a blender.
2. Apply to freshly cleaned face and leave on for 15 minutes.
3. Wash off with warm water and pat dry.

The acid in the tomato and lemon work on acne and blackheads.

Hydrating mask

Ingredients:
20 g of yeast
yogurt

Instructions:
1. Dissolve 20 g yeast small amount of yogurt to the consistency of thick cream.
2. Apply on clean skin for 15-20 minutes.
3. Rinse with warm water and dried up mask.

Peach mask

Ingredients:
1 medium peach
1 tablespoons honey
Oatmeal

Instructions:
1. Cook peach until its soft, mash with a fork, add honey and oatmeal until it's a thick consistency.
2. Apply on the face for 10 minutes.
3. Rinse well with cool water.

Raspberry mask

Ingredients:
Puree raspberries
1 teaspoon of honey

Instructions:
1. Mix 2 tablespoons of the pure with one teaspoon of honey.
2. Apply on face for about 15 minutes. If mixture turns out to be too fluid and runny, put it on a piece of gauze and then apply to face.

You can use this refreshing mask two or three times a week. It is especially good for the hot summer months.

Combination Skin Type Masks

Combination skin type care is difficult and troublesome. Its peculiarity consists in the fact that several types of preparations for different facial parts must be combined. With the combination skin type it is usually the chin, nose (especially the wings) and the centre of the forehead which are oily while the cheeks and the neck are dry. In this case you should apply a purifying mask to the central part of your face and moisturizing or nutritious masks for the other parts.

Before applying the masks you should moisten the centre of the face with tepid water and put some moisturizing cream on the cheeks and neck.

Purifying Honey Mask with Aloe Vera

Ingredients:
Aloe Vera 1pcs
Bean curd or Tofu half
1 teaspoon of honey

Instructions:
1. Clean the Aloe Vera with water, remove the Aloe Vera peel.
2. Put the Aloe Vera flesh and bean curd or Tofu to into a mixer and blend until it mix well.
3. Extract the juice with pledget.
4. Add in honey into the Bean curd and aloe Vera juice, stir until it fully disolved.
5. After facial cleansing, gently smear this Aloe Vera Honey mask on the face (avoiding eye and lip area).
6. Leave it for 15 minutes.
7. Wash with warm water.

Clay Mask

Ingredients:
1½ teaspoon of green clay (French is preferred)
½ teaspoon of kaolin clay

1½ teaspoon of Aloe Vera gel
1 tablespoon of rosewater
2 drops of rose essential oil

Instructions:
1. Mix green and kaolin clays together.
2. Add in the Aloe Vera gel, rosewater and oils.
3. Apply on the face on for 10-15 minutes.
4. Wash with warm water.
Refrigerate mixture for up to four weeks.

Honey mask with blackcurrant

Ingredients:
1 tablespoon of honey
2 tablespoons of blackcurrant juice

Instructions:
1. Steam-melt honey and add blackcurrant juice. Mix well.
2. Apply mask on the face and neck area for 30 minutes.
3. Rinse away with cool water.

Egg mask with blackcurrant

Ingredients:
1 egg white
1 tablespoon of blackcurrant juice

Instructions:
1. Mix egg white with the blackcurrant juice.
2. Apply on the face, wash off after 10 minutes.
You can use a mask every 3 days.

Cucumber Mask

Ingredients:
1 tablespoon of nonfat dry milk
1 egg white

1/2 peeled cucumber
1 teaspoon of plain yogurt
1 teaspoon of mint

Instructions:
1. Blend all these ingredients in a blender until smooth and well mixed.
2. Apply on the face with a foundation brush.
3. Put a slice of cucumber on each eye and relax for 20 min.
4. Rinse with water.

Herbal mask

Ingredients:
1 egg
1/2 cup of oatmeal
1 teaspoon of olive oil

Instructions:
1. Mix 1 egg with 1/2 cup of cooked instant oatmeal.
2. Put in 1 teaspoon of olive oil (or more if your skin needs a little extra hydration).
3. Leave this mask on the face for 15 minutes.
4. Rinse with warm water.
Your skin should be toned and radiant.

Apple mask

Ingredients:
1/2 of an apple
1 tablespoon of warm milk
1 egg yolk
1 tablespoon of pure oatmeal(optional, but recommended)

Instructions:
1. Puree the apple in a food processor, blender, or any other appliance used for pureeing food. (Leaving the peel on is optional.)
2. Add the warm milk and mix until blended.

3. Add the egg yolk and break it a bit, then mix it in, binding all three ingredients together.

4. If you see that your mixture is a bit too runny, add a bit of oatmeal to make it more spreadable.

5. Apply on your face for 10-15 minutes. Using the back curved part of a spoon is the easiest way.

6. Wash off with warm water.

7. Pat dry with a towel.

Yoghurt mask

Ingredients:
100 grams of natural yoghurt
1 egg-white

Instructions:
1. Mix 100 grams of natural yoghurt with an egg-white.
2. Apply on the face fro 15-20 minutes.
3. Wash the mask with warm water.

Rye-bread mask

Ingredients:
Rye-bread
1 tablespoon of honey
25 grams of milk

Instructions:
1. Mix a round of rye-bread with a tablespoon of honey and 25 grams of warm milk.
2. Apply on the face for 20 minutes.
3. Wash off with warm water.

Curds mask

Ingredients:
2 tablespoons of curds
1 tablespoon of milk
Salt

1 tablespoon of olive oil

Instructions:
1. Mix two tablespoons of rich curds with a tablespoon of warm milk
2. Add a bit of salt and a tablespoon of olive oil.
3. Mix all these ingredients.
4. Apply the mask on your face for 15-20 minutes.
5. Wash off with warm water.

Sandalwood and Milk mask

Ingredients:
1 tablespoon of sandalwood powder
Milk

Instructions:
1. Take one tablespoon of sandalwood powder and enough milk to make a paste.
This mask is removes excess heat from the skin and cools the skin.

Honey and Oatmeal Mask

Ingredients:
2 tablespoons of honey
2 teaspoons of oatmeal

Instructions:
1. Take 2 tablespoons of honey and 2 teaspoons of oatmeal.
2. Mix and apply on the face for 20 minutes.
3. Wash off with cold water.
This is perfect face mask as it hydrates the skin and removes dead skin.

Yogurt and Mint mask

Ingredients:
1 tablespoon of yogurt

2 teaspoons of mint juice

Instructions:
1. Take 1 tablespoon of yogurt and 2 teaspoons of mint juice.
2. Mix and apply on the face.
3. Wash off with cold water.

Yogurt is great for skin it gives an instant glow to the skin and makes it soft and supple.

Banana with Avocado Mask

Ingredients:
1/2 banana
1/2 avocado
2 tablespoons of full-fat yogurt
1 teaspoon of olive oil

Instructions:
1. Puree all ingredients in a blender.
2. Apply to freshly cleaned face and leave on for 15 minutes.
3. Wash off with warm water and pat dry.

Papaya Mask

Ingredients:
1 papaya

Instructions:
1. Peel and remove seeds. Chop into pieces and drop into food processor.
2. Puree until papaya is the consistancy of baby food.
3. Use 1/2 a tablespoon for each facial. Keep leftovers in a baggie in the frig.

Mask contains a strong enzyme called papain which dissolves oil and dead skin cells.

Cornmeal Facial Scrub

Ingredients:

Cornmeal
Water

Instructions:
1. Mix cornmeal with enough water to make a paste.
2. Apply on the face in a circular motion.
3. Allow to dry and rinse off with cool water.

Rose facial mask

Ingredients:
The crushed petals from one rose
1 tablespoon of yogurt and honey
1 tablespoon of rosewater
1 tablespoon of honey

Instructions:
1. Mix all the ingredients and apply it on the face with gentle circular massage motions.
2. Rinse the mask off after 15 minutes.

Normal Skin Type Masks

Normal skin type is very rare and does not require special care. Still, to save this natural gift, you should take certain care of it.

Normal skin type should be cleaned, nourished and kept protected from the deleterious effects of the environment. We recommend you to use the following masks.

Carrot mask with olive oil

Ingredients:
1 tablespoon of carrot juice
1 egg yolk
1/2 teaspoons of olive oil

Instructions:
1. Mix carrot juice and egg yolks, add the olive oil and pound.
2. Apply on the face for 10 minutes
3. Wash off with warm water.

Strawberry Mask

Ingredients:
½ cup ripe strawberries
¼ cup cornstarch

Instructions:
1. Mix the cornstarch and strawberries.
2. Apply the mask on the face. Avoid the eye area as strawberries can be quiet acidic.
3. Leave it on for about 30 minutes.
4. Rinse with cool water.
This will help you freshen up and vitalize your face.

Honey and apple mask

Ingredients:
1 apple

2 tablespoons of honey

Instructions:
1. Skin an apple and cut it into pieces.
2. Blend it in a food processor with 2 tablespoons of honey.
3. Apply the mixture on your face in a circular motion.
4. Leave it for 30 minutes before rinsing.

This mask gives your skin a refreshed and cared-for look.

Parsley Honey Face Mask

Ingredients:
2 tablespoons of parsley
1 egg yolk
1 tablespoon of honey

Instructions:
1. Blend the parsley with the egg yolk and then add honey.
2. Apply the mask to your clean face and relax for 20 minutes.
3. Rinse it off.

Parsley-Carrot Mask

Ingredients:
1/4 cup of fresh carrot juice
1/4 cup of white clay
1 teaspoon of fresh parsley

Instructions:
1. Mix together all ingredients until you have a smooth, creamy mixture.
2. Apply the mask on clean skin using your fingertips or a small brush.
3. Leave it on for about 20 minutes.
4. Rinse it well with warm water followed by cool water. Pat skin dry.

Store any remaining mask in the refrigerator for up to 1 week.

Flax-Seeds

Ingredients:
2 tablespoons of grounded flax-seeds
4 tablespoons of hot mineral water

Instructions:
1. Add 2 tablespoons of grounded flax-seeds to 4 tablespoons of hot mineral water and mix it carefully.
2. Cover the glass with the mixture and leave it to cool down.

Cream mask

Ingredients:
1/2 cup of cream
2-3 teaspoons of wheat flour

Instructions:
1. Mix cream and flour.
2. Apply the mask on the face.
3. Allow to dry.
4. Rinse the face well with warm water.

Chamomile Honey Mask

Ingredients:
113g of clear honey
15g of dried chamomile flowers
10 drops of Chamomile Roman essential oil

Instructions:
1. Place the honey into a double boiler or bain marie and heat gently until melted.
2. Stir in the chamomile flowers.
3. Cover with a lid and leave on the lowest heat for thirty minutes.
4. Remove from the heat and allow the chamomile flowers to soak in the honey for two hours.
5. Strain through a fine sieve and pour into a clean, dark glass jar.

6. Drop in the chamomile essential oil and stir well to combine.

7. Apply lightly on the face and neck after cleansing.

8. Leave on for twenty minutes and then rinse with lukewarm water.

Cucumber Mask

Ingredients:
1 tablespoon unsalted butter, softened
1 inch slice of cucumber, chopped and mashed

Instructions:
1. Beat both the above ingredients together.
2. Apply on the face for 10 minutes.
3. Wash face with lukewarm water.
4. Pat your face dry with a soft towel.

Green Honey Face Mask

Ingredients:
1 medium banana
3 tablespoons honey
2 egg whites
4 cups fresh spinach; rinsed
1 cup mint; rinsed
1-inch ginger; peeled

Instructions:
1. Pulse ingredients in a blender until cut up and then blend until smooth.

2. Add the banana and the honey and continue to blend the ingredients until it is liquidy.

3. Add the egg whites and blend.

4. Apply on the face and neck avoiding the eye area.

5. Leave on your face for 15 minutes.

6. Rinse off facial mask with warm water.

Honey mask with vodka

Ingredients:
100 g of honey
50 grams of vodka

Instructions:
1. Mix honey well with vodka.
2. Apply the mask on the face for 10 - 15 minutes.
3. Rinse with warm water.
This mask disinfects and softens the skin.

Honey Lemon Mask

Ingredients:
1/2 of a real lemon or a few drops of lemon oil (it has the same effect)
2 teaspoons of honey

Instructions:
1. Squeeze 1/2 of the lemon into a bowl, mix in honey and stir until its like cough syrup.
2. Apply mask to freshly cleansed face for about 20 minutes and try not to talk. Make sure you don't exfoliate your skin before adding this mask because the lemon juice can make it sting.
3. Rinse off with cold water and pat dry your face.

You can do this every morning or every night.

Mustard mask

Ingredients:
1/2 cup of mustard
2 liters of water

Instructions:
1. Take 1/2 cup of mustard and grind it in two liters of water.
2. Make a paste of it with some rose petals.
3. Apply it on the face for half an hour.
4. Wash it off.

Peachy mask

Ingredients:
1 medium peach
1 tablespoon of honey
1 tablespoon of oatmeal

Instructions:
1. Cook peach until its soft, mash with a fork.
2. Add honey and oatmeal until it is a thick consistency.
3. Apply on the face for 10 minutes.
4. Rinse well with cool water.

Yeast mask

Ingredients:
10 g of yeast
2 tablespoons of milk

Instructions:
1. Mix a bit of fresh yeast with milk until the consistency of sour cream.
2. Apply to the skin for 10-15 minutes.
3. Rinse first with hot then cold water.

With regular use of this mask the skin becomes clear and matte.

Egg-lemon mask

Ingredients:
1 egg white
1 teaspoon of lemon juice
Salt - to the tip of a knife.

Instructions:
1. Beat the white of one egg.
2. Add lemon juice and a pinch of fine salt.
3. Apply the foam on the face for 15-20 minutes.

4. Rinse with warm water.

Egg mask with glycerol

Ingredients:
1 egg white
1 teaspoon of lemon juice
1 teaspoon of glycerin
1 teaspoon of vegetable oil

Instructions:
1. Beat the white of one egg with lemon juice.
2. Add the glycerin and vegetable oil.
3. Apply on the face for 10 minutes.
4. Rinse with warm water.

Oatmeal Mask with Honey

Ingredients:
1/3 cup of fast cook oatmeal (1-3 minutes)
¼ cup of honey
½ cup of water

Instructions:
1. Mix the water and the oatmeal together, and cook.
2. Set the oatmeal aside to cool and thicken.
3. As it is cooling, mix in the ¼ cup of honey.
4. Apply a on the face for 20 minutes.
5. Rinse with warm water.

Herbal mask

Ingredients:
Leaves of mint, lemon balm, plantain and calendula flowers in equal parts
1/2 cup of water

Instructions:

1. Chop the leaves of mint, lemon balm, plantain, calendula flowers.

2. Pour a small amount of boiling water to get porridge. Let stand in a sealed container.

3. Place porridge on the gauze and apply on the face.

Rose mask

Ingredients:
1 teaspoon of sour cream
1 teaspoon of honey
1 teaspoon of crushed rose petals

Instructions:
1. Mix sour cream with honey and add the rose petals.
2. Apply to clean skin for 20 minutes.
3. Rinse with warm water.

Raw potatoes mask

Ingredients:
1 potato

Instructions:
1. Grate raw potatoes.
2. Apply on the face.
3. Leave it on for 15-20 minutes.
4. Rinse with warm water.

Kiwi mask

Ingredients:
1 kiwi
1 tablespoon of honey
1 tablespoon of raw lemon juice

Instructions:
1. Blend one kiwi with 1 teaspoon of raw honey and 1 teaspoon lemon juice.

2. Apply to clean, dry skin.

3. Leave the mask on for 20 minutes.
4. Rinse off with warm water.

Apricot mask

Ingredients:
3-4 large apricots
1 teaspoon of oatmeal or wheat flour

Instructions:
1. Rub apricots with oatmeal or wheat flour.
2. Apply on face for 15 minutes.
3. Wash off with non-carbonated mineral water.

Masks for Dry Skin Type

Facial masks are usually divided into nutritious, cleanser and moisturizing but, as a rule, each mask contains all three components, one of them prevailing.

Dry and sensitive skin type facial masks should be selected very carefully as the result can be reverse to what was expected. Before applying the masks read through the list of ingredients and ensure that none of them make your skin irritated.

Egg and honey hydrating facial mask

Ingredients:
1 egg
1/4 cup of coconut oil
1 teaspoon of honey

Instructions:
1. Scramble the egg and gradually add honey and coconut oil. The mass should look like mayonnaise. If it is too thick, add more coconut oil. If it is too runny, add a bit more honey.
2. Pour the mass into a plastic cup, close the cup tightly, and leave in the fridge overnight.
3. This mask is ready to be applied the next day. Scoop up some of the mask and freely apply all over the face.
4. Leave it to rest for 10 minutes.
5. Wash off with lukewarm water.

Cucumber and olive oil mask

Ingredients:
3 cucumbers very finely diced
3 teaspoons of olive oil
2 teaspoons of live yogurt

Instructions:
1. Mix above ingredients into a fine paste.
2. Leave to dry for about 15 minutes.
3. Wash off with cold water.

Skin feels soft, conditioned and clean.

Honey Mask

Ingredients:
1 raw egg
1 tablespoon of honey

Instructions:
1. Mix together egg and honey.
2. Apply on the face for 15-20 minutes.
3. Rinse well with tepid water.

Yogurt and Aloe Vera Mask

Ingredients:
1 egg yellow
1 tablespoon of Aloe Vera Juice
1 tablespoon of organic Yogurt
½ spoon of sunflower oil

Instructions:
1. Stir the ingredients.
2. Apply on the face for 15 minutes.
3. Wash off with morerate-temperature water.
Use it up to twice a week.

Aloe Vera and Honey Mask

Ingredients:
2 spoons of honey, slightly heated
1 tblespoon of orange juice
1 tablespoon of Aloe Vera juice
Instructions:
1. Mix all ingredients.
2. Apply on the for 15 minutes
3. Wash off with lukewarm water.

This mask has a smoothing effect and prevents an appearance of wrinkles.

Avocado mask

Ingredients:
1 ripe avocado
1 egg yolk
1/2 teaspoon of olive oil
1/2 teaspoon of almond oil

Instructions:
1. In a blender blitz all the ingredients together until you have a smooth consistency.
2. Apply on the face.
3. Leave on for about 15 minutes.
4. Rinse off with tepid water.

Soothing Clay Mask

Ingredients:
1 ounce red or white clay
3 tablespoons of rose water
1 teaspoon of jojoba
2 drops of Chamomile essential oil
2 drops of Rose essential oil

Instructions:
1. Combine the clay and the floral or distilled water in a bowl and mix well until a good thick paste is formed.
2. Add the remaining ingredients and mix well.
3. Apply on a clean, damp face. Avoid the eye area for 15 minutes.
4. Rinse off well with warm water.

Avocado and Olive Oil Mask

Ingredients:
1/2 avocado
1 tablespoon of olive oil

Instructions:
1. Mash the avocado and the olive oil together in a bowl.
2. Apply to your face for 20 minutes.
3. Rinse with warm water.

Chocolate Mask

Ingredients:
1 tablespoon of cocoa powder
1 tablespoon of heavy cream
1 teaspoon of cottage cheese
4 teaspoons of honey
1 teaspoon of oatmeal

Instructions:
1. Puree all ingredients in a blender.
2. Apply on freshly cleaned face for 10 minutes.
3. Wash off with warm water and pat dry.

Egyptian Mask

1 whole egg
1/2 teaspoon of olive oil
1 tablespoon of flour
1/4 teaspoon of sea salt
1 tablespoon of whole milk

Instructions:
1. Beat the egg in a small bowl. In a large bowl mix together the all of the ingredients, stirring in the sea salt last.
2. Apply on the face and neck in a light circular motion avoiding the eye area.
3. Leave on for 15 minutes.
4. Rinse off this facial mask with lukewarm water, following with cold water.

Berries and Cream Facial Mask

Ingredients:
7 tablespoons of thick cream
3-5 strawberries
3-5 any other berries of your choice
2 teaspoons of honey

Instructions:
1. In a bowl whip the cream until peaks start to form.
2. In another bowl mash in the strawberries and honey together.
3. Fold in the cream mixture into the strawberries and mix it all together until it's blended well.
4. Apply on the face for about 20-30 minutes.
5. Rinse off with warm water.

Moisturizing berry mask

Ingredients:
2-3 raspberries
2-3 strawberries
1 apricot
1 teaspoon of grated fresh cabbage
1 teaspoon cream

Instructions:
1. Mash all berries and mix them.
2. Add the cabbage and cream.
3. Apply on the face for 15 minutes.
4. Rinse off with cool water and then warm and then cool.

Toning curd Mask

Ingredients:
2 teaspoons of fat cottage cheese
2 teaspoons of milk
2 teaspoons of fresh carrot juice

Instructions:
1. Mash cottage cheese, milk and carrot juice.

2. Apply on face for 20 minutes and then remove it from the face

3. Wash off the remains of the mask with a solution of cucumber infusion and decoction of chamomile.

Banana Oatmeal Mask

Ingredients:
1/2 cup of cooked oatmeal
1 teaspoon of honey
1 egg yolk
1/2 banana, mashed

Instructions:
1. Combine all ingredients.
2. Apply on the face for 15 minutes.
3. Rise off with cool water.

Orange Cleansing Mask

Ingredients:
1 egg yolk
2 teaspoons of orange juice
1/2 teaspoon of honey
1/2 teaspoon of almond oil

Instructions:
1. Beat the egg yolk and orange juice together with a fork. Continue beating the mixture until the yolk is creamy in texture.

2. Add the honey and then the almond oil, beating well after each addition.

3. Apply the mask on the face for a 1/2 hour. Avoid the sensitive skin around your eyes.

4. Rinse off with cool water.

Watermelons and papaya mask

Ingredients:
1/2 Watermelon
2 small pieces of Papaya

1 Banana
A little Milk Cream

Instructions:
1. Take some steam on face.
2. Mix the watermelon, papaya, banana and cream into a paste.
3. Apply it on face for 15-20 minutes and massage.
4. Wash with cold water.

Brown Sugar and Milk Mask

Ingredients:
1/4 cup of brown sugar
1 - 2 tablespoons of milk

Instructions:
1. Mix the all ingredients.
2. Apply to freshly cleaned face and massage gently for a full minute.
3. Leave on for 15 minutes.
4. Wash off with warm water and pat dry.

Rosewood Exfoliating Mask

Ingredients:
2 tablespoons of sugar
3 tablespoons of warm water
2 drops of essential oil - rosewood

Instructions:
1. Stir sugar in warm water until dissolved.
2. Add rosewood essential oil.
3. Apply to freshly cleaned face and massage gently for 5 minutes.
4. Wash off with warm water and pat dry.

This mask is excellent for exfoliating dead skin.

Avocado and Honey Face Mask

Ingredients:
2 tablespoons of avocado flesh
2 tablespoons honey
1 egg yolk

Instructions:
1. Put all the ingredients in a blender, or mash by hand in a bowl.
2. Use your fingers to spread the mask over the face for at least 30 minutes, preferably longer, before removing.

Lavender and Honey Facial Mask

Ingredients:
3 drops of lavender oil (not fragrance oil)
1 tablespoon of honey

Instructions:
1. Combine the honey and lavender in a small bowl. Stir until mixed well.
2. Apply on the face with your fingertips for 10 to 15 minutes, then rinse well.
3. Wash your face with your usual skin cleanser.